# Feel and look 30 years younger

# Hazel Summers

# Table of contents

# Introduction



The motivation behind this book is to give an exhaustive aide on the most proficient method to look 30 years more youthful and keep a sound, solid, and long life. The book will cover different parts of taking care of oneself, including healthy skin, work out, diet, rest, stress of the executives, cosmetics and preparation, and way of life changes. The objective is to give readers the information and devices they need to carry out certain progressions in their lives and accomplish their wellbeing and excellence objectives. Through the book, readers will find out about the significance of dealing with themselves, both all around, and the job that different elements play in the aging system. The motivation behind the book is to enable readers to pursue informed decisions and take on an all encompassing way to deal with their prosperity.

# Skin care

A fundamental skin health management routine can be broken down into the accompanying advances:

<u>Exfoliate</u>:
Begin by purging your face with a delicate chemical that is reasonable for your skin type. This will assist with eliminating soil, oil, and cosmetics, leaving your skin feeling invigorated and clean.

<u>Tone</u>:
Utilize a toner to assist with adjusting the skin's pH and eliminate any lingering debasements. Conditioning likewise assists with setting up the skin for the subsequent stages in your daily practice.

<u>Treat</u>:

Apply any medicines or serums that you use to target explicit skin concerns, like dim spots, scarcely discernible differences, or kinks.

Moisturize:
Wrap up by applying a cream to assist with hydrating the skin and lock in dampness. This will assist with forestalling dryness and keep the skin feeling delicate and flexible.

Sun protection:
Remember to apply a wide range sunscreen with essentially SPF 30 to shield your skin from harmful UV beams.

It's essential that everybody's skin is unique, and what works for one individual may not work for another. It might take an experimentation to track down the right items and routine for your skin, however with just enough tolerance and determination, you can accomplish sound, sparkling skin. Moreover, it's essential to be delicate with your skin and try not to utilize cruel items that can cause bother or harm.

# How to cope with specific skin concerns

With regards to treating explicit skin concerns, for example, skin inflammation or hyperpigmentation, it's critical to utilize items that are customized to your singular requirements. For instance, on the off chance that you have skin break out inclined skin, you might need to utilize a salicylic corrosive based chemical or a benzoyl peroxide spot treatment to assist with clearing up breakouts. Assuming you have hyperpigmentation, you might need to utilize an item containing fixings like L-ascorbic acid or kojic corrosive, which can assist with lighting up the skin and, surprisingly, out complexion.

It's likewise critical to talk with a dermatologist or skincare expert to get a legitimate conclusion and suggestions on the best items and fixings to use for your particular skin concerns. They can likewise assist with making a customized healthy skin schedule that will give you the best outcomes.

It's critical to take note of that while a few over-the-counter items can be successful, original potency drugs and medicines might be required for more serious or persevering skin concerns. A dermatologist can likewise screen your skin and change your daily schedule on a case by case basis to guarantee that you obtain the best outcomes.

## Anti-aging skin care products

Indeed, consolidating hostile to aging items, like retinol or hyaluronic corrosive, into your skincare routine can assist with dialing back the aging system and keep a young appearance.

Retinol is a type of vitamin A that is generally perceived for its enemy of aging properties. It works by expanding cell turnover and advancing collagen creation, which assists with lessening the presence of scarce differences and kinks, and further develops skin surface and tone.

Hyaluronic corrosive is a characteristic substance that is tracked down in the skin and assists with keeping it hydrated and stout. As we age, our body's normal degrees of hyaluronic corrosive decline, prompting dryness and kinks. By utilizing items that contain hyaluronic corrosiveness, you can assist with supporting your skin's hydration levels and re-establish an energetic, full appearance.

The utilization of hostile to aging items can be exceptionally individual and rely upon your skin type, concerns, and objectives. It's ideal to talk with a skincare expert or dermatologist to decide the best items and fixings to use for your particular requirements. Also, it means quite a bit to utilize these items as coordinated, and to be patient and predictable with their utilization, as the outcomes may not be prompt.

# Importance of a daily skin care routine

An everyday skin health management routine is significant for keeping up with sound and energetic looking skin. A decent skin health management routine assists with keeping the skin perfect, hydrated, and shielded from ecological stressors that can cause harm and untimely aging. An everyday healthy skin routine likewise assists with keeping up with the skin's normal obstruction capability, which assists with forestalling dampness, misfortune, bothering, and the entrance of unsafe substances.

Likewise, an everyday healthy skin routine can assist with working on the presence of skin blemishes, like scarcely discernible differences, wrinkles, dim spots, and bluntness. By integrating the right items and methods into your everyday practice, you can assist with reestablishing the skin's regular sparkle and immovability, while additionally tending to explicit skin worries that you might have. A day to day skin health management routine is a straightforward and compelling method for putting resources into your skin's wellbeing and prosperity, and can have dependable advantages for your general appearance and self-assurance.

## Importance of using products that are suitable for your skin type

Utilizing items that are reasonable for your skin type is fundamental for accomplishing solid, sparkling skin. Different skin types, like slick, dry, blend, or delicate, have various necessities and concerns, and require various items to keep up with ideal wellbeing and appearance.

For instance, those with sleek skin might profit from utilizing lightweight, sans oil items that won't obstruct pores, while those with dry skin might require seriously feeding, hydrating items to assist with keeping up with dampness levels. Those with irritating skin might profit from utilizing delicate, scent free items that will not aggravate or cause redness.

Utilizing items that are not reasonable for your skin type can prompt skin aggravation, breakouts, and different issues, like dryness or slickness. Moreover, utilizing items that are excessively cruel or not compelling for your skin type can prompt an absence of progress or improvement in your skin concerns.

To decide your skin type, it's vital to consider factors like sleekness, dryness, awareness, and the presence of explicit skin concerns, like skin inflammation or dull spots. You can likewise talk with a skincare expert or dermatologist to get a legitimate determination and proposals on the best items and fixings to use for your particular skin type.

All in all, utilizing items that are appropriate for your skin type is significant for accomplishing solid, gleaming skin and keeping up with the outcomes after some time.

# Skin care kits to avoid

While picking skincare items, it's essential to be aware of specific healthy skin packs that may not be viable or appropriate for your skin type and concerns. Some skin health management units to keep away from include:

- One-size-fits-all units:

Some healthy skin packs are promoted as "one-size-fits-all" and vow to work for all skin types. Be that as it may, each skin is one of a kind, and what works for one individual may not work for another. It's critical to pick items that are customized to your singular skin type and concerns.

- Units with cruel fixings:

Some healthy skin packs contain brutal fixings, for example, high convergences of acids or peeling specialists, that can aggravate or harm the skin whenever utilized inappropriately. Be aware of the fixings in any healthy skin unit you consider, and pick items that are delicate and appropriate for your skin type.

- Overrated units:

Some healthy skin packs are evaluated altogether higher than comparative items sold independently. It's vital to be aware of the expense of any healthy skin pack and pick items that are sensibly evaluated and offer great incentive for cash.

- Units with sketchy cases:

Some healthy skin packs make misrepresented or problematic cases, for example, promising to delete barely recognizable differences and kinks in a short measure of time. Have misgivings of any skin health management unit that causes guarantees that to appear to be unrealistic, and pick items that have a strong history of conveying results.

All in all, it's essential to be careful while picking healthy skin packs, and to pick items that are customized to your singular skin type and concerns, are delicate, sensibly evaluated, and have a strong history of conveying results.

# Exercise

Practice assumes a significant part in keeping up with sound skin and an energetic appearance. Standard actual work has a few advantages for the skin, including:

#1. Further developed course: Exercise increments blood stream, which assists with carrying oxygen and supplements to the skin and advance cell development. Further developed dissemination additionally assists with eliminating poisons from the skin, keeping it solid and sparkling.

#2. Expanded collagen creation: Collagen is a protein that gives the skin its versatility and immovability. Normal activity can expand the creation of collagen, assisting with keeping the skin looking energetic and lessening the presence of scarce differences and kinks.

#3. Decreased stress: Stress can adversely affect the skin, causing breakouts, redness, and bluntness. Practice is a compelling method for diminishing stress and advance unwinding, which can assist with working on the presence of the skin.

#4. Better sleep: Exercise can likewise assist with working on the nature of rest, which is fundamental for solid skin. At the point when we rest, our bodies work to fix and revive the skin, so getting sufficient tranquil rest is critical for keeping a young appearance.

#5. Hydration: Exercise increases sweat creation, which assists with hydrating the skin and flushing out poisons. It's essential to remain hydrated by drinking water previously, during, and after exercise to keep up with sound skin.

The sort and power of activity that is best for your skin will rely upon your singular requirements and objectives. It's ideal to talk with a specialist or wellness expert to decide the best work-out everyday practice for you.

Standard exercise assumes a vital part in keeping up with solid skin and a young appearance. Exercise can assist you with accomplishing and keeping up with sound, sparkling skin.

## Types of exercise to incorporate

There are a wide range of
kinds of activity that can be integrated into a daily schedule to keep up with solid skin and an energetic appearance. The absolute most advantageous sorts of activity for the skin include:

1. Oxygen consuming activity: High-impact workout, like running, cycling, or swimming, can further develop course, increment collagen creation, and decrease stress. These kinds of activities can assist with keeping the skin looking solid and brilliant.

2. Strength preparing: Strength preparing, like weightlifting or bodyweight works out, can assist with expanding bulk and work on bone thickness, which can assist with keeping the skin looking firm and young.

3. Yoga: Yoga is a delicate type of activity that joins actual development with care and breathing procedures. It can assist with decreasing stress, further develop course, and advance unwinding, all of which can help the skin.

4. Outside work out: Investing energy in the outside air and daylight can assist with helping the skin's normal vitamin D creation, which is significant for solid skin. Outside work out, like climbing, planting, or playing sports, can likewise assist with further developing flow and decrease stress.

5. Stop and go aerobic exercise (HIIT): HIIT is a kind of activity that includes short explosions of extreme action followed by times of rest. This

kind of activity can assist with expanding course, help collagen creation, and diminish stress, all of which can help the skin.

It's vital that the kind and power of activity that is best for your skin will rely upon your singular requirements and objectives. Integrating a wide range of activities into your routine can assist with keeping up with sound skin and an energetic appearance. High-impact workout, strength preparing, yoga, open air work out, and HIIT are powerful methods for further developing flow, increment collagen creation, decrease stress, and lift the skin's wellbeing and appearance.

## Importance of finding an exercise routine you enjoy

Finding a work-out schedule that is charming and economical is urgent for keeping up with sound skin and an energetic appearance. There are a few justifications for why finding a work-out schedule that you appreciate and can adhere to is significant:

-Expanded adherence: When you partake in your work-out daily schedule, you're bound to adhere to it. On the off chance that you're abhorring your activity, you're bound to skip exercises or quit altogether, which can adversely influence the wellbeing of your skin.

-Decreased stress: Exercise is intended to diminish stress, not cause it. On the off chance that you're despising your work-out daily schedule, it can really increase stress, which can adversely affect the skin.

-Good on emotional well-being: Exercise is additionally significant for keeping up with great psychological wellness. At the point when you partake in your work-out daily schedule, it can assist with helping your state of mind and decrease uneasiness, which can help the skin.

-Improved results: When you partake in your work-out everyday practice, you're bound to stay with it and see improved results. Whether you're attempting to work on your course, increment collagen creation, or decrease stress, finding an agreeable work-out routine can assist you with accomplishing your objectives.

The kind of activity that is agreeable for you will rely upon your singular inclinations and objectives. Certain individuals appreciate extreme focus exercises, while others favor low-influence exercises like yoga or strolling. It's ideal to try different things with various kinds of activity to find what you appreciate and what turns out best for your skin.

At the point when you partake in your work-out daily practice, you're bound to adhere to it, lessen stress, work on emotional wellness, and see improved results, all of which can help the wellbeing and presence of your skin.

# Facial exercises

Integrating facial activities into your day to day schedule can assist with conditioning and fix the muscles in front of you, giving your skin a more energetic and lifted appearance. The absolute best facial activities for conditioning and fixing include:

-Brow wrinkles: This exercise includes utilizing your fingertips to apply delicate strain to your temple while you scrunch your eyebrows together. This can assist with fortifying and tone the muscles in your brow.

-Cheek lifts: To perform cheek lifts, just grin as wide as possible while lifting your cheeks towards your eyes. This exercise can assist with conditioning the muscles in your cheeks and give your face a more lifted appearance.

-Jaw grasps: This exercise includes gripping your jaw and standing firm on the footing for a few seconds. It can assist with conditioning and fix the muscles in your jaw and neck.

-Lip sulks: To perform lip frowns, just mop your lips as though you were going to blow a kiss. This exercise can assist with conditioning the muscles around your mouth and forestall the arrangement of barely recognizable differences and kinks.

-Eye crushes: This exercise includes shutting your eyes firmly and standing firm on the footing for a few seconds. It can assist with conditioning the muscles around your eyes and forestall the arrangement of crow's feet.

These facial activities ought to be performed delicately and with alertness, as exaggerating them can prompt muscle strain and inconvenience. It's ideal to begin with only a couple of redundancies of each activity and continuously increment the quantity of reiterations as your muscles get more grounded.

# Dieting

Diet assumes a significant part in keeping up with solid skin. The food varieties you eat can affect the wellbeing of your skin in more than one way, including:

**Hydration**:
Drinking a lot of water is fundamental for keeping your skin hydrated and looking solid. Dried out skin can look dull and dormant, and can be more defenseless to kinks and scarce differences.

**Supplement consumption**: Eating an eating routine that is plentiful in nutrients, minerals, and cell reinforcements can assist with supporting the strength of your skin. Nutrients C and E, for instance, are significant for safeguarding your skin from harm brought about by free revolutionaries, while vitamin A is urgent for keeping up with the wellbeing of your skin cells.

**Irritation**:

An eating routine that is high in handled and sweet food varieties can aggravate aggravation in your body, which can harm your skin cells and make your skin more defenseless to aging and wrinkles. Eating an eating regimen that is wealthy in mitigating food sources, like salad greens, berries, and greasy fish, can assist with decreasing irritation and backing the soundness of your skin.

**Hormonal equilibrium**:

A few food varieties can influence your chemicals and add to skin issues, like skin inflammation or dermatitis. Eating an eating regimen that is adjusted and incorporates a lot of new foods grown from the ground can assist with keeping up with hormonal equilibrium and backing the soundness of your skin.

It's essential that everybody's skin and dietary requirements are one of a kind, so it's ideal to work with a dermatologist or nutritionist to decide the best eating routine for your skin.

Drinking a lot of water, eating an eating routine that is plentiful in nutrients, minerals, and cell reinforcements, decreasing irritation, and keeping up with hormonal equilibrium are terrifically significant elements that can influence the wellbeing and presence of your skin.

## Recommendations for a healthy diet

A sound eating regimen can emphatically affect your skin wellbeing, as well as your general wellbeing and prosperity. Here are a few proposals for a solid eating regimen:

-Incorporate a lot of foods grown from the ground: Expect to eat something like five parts of products of the soil each day, as they are plentiful in nutrients, minerals, and cell reinforcements that are fundamental for solid skin.

-Eat lean protein: Lean protein sources, like chicken, fish, and vegetables, are significant for keeping up with sound skin and supporting the development of new skin cells.

-Pick whole grains: whole grain food sources, like earthy colored rice, whole wheat bread, and oats, are an extraordinary wellspring of fiber and can assist with keeping up with stable glucose levels, which is significant for sound skin.

-Incorporate sound fats: Food varieties that are high in solid fats, like avocados, nuts, and greasy fish, can assist with keeping your skin hydrated and decrease aggravation.

-Limit processed and sweet food sources: Processed and sweet food sources can increase irritation and add to skin issues, like skin inflammation and untimely aging. It's ideal to restrict your admission of these food sources and pick better choices all things being equal.

-Remain hydrated: Drinking a lot of water is fundamental for keeping your skin hydrated and sound. Expect to drink something like 8 glasses of water each day.

It's essential that everybody's dietary requirements are unique, and it's ideal to work with a nutritionist to decide the best eating regimen for your particular necessities and objectives.

## When to adjust your diet

Paying attention to your body and changing your eating routine case by case is essential for keeping up with ideal skin wellbeing. Our bodies are continually changing and adjusting, and our dietary necessities can change thus. Here are a few motivations behind why it's vital to pay attention to your body and change your eating routine on a case by case basis:

-Food awareness: Certain individuals might foster aversions to specific food sources over the long run, and these responsive qualities can influence their skin wellbeing. For instance, consuming dairy items or gluten might cause skin irritation and breakouts in certain people.

-Hormonal changes: Hormonal changes, for example, during a period or pregnancy, can influence your dietary necessities and skin wellbeing. For instance, you might have to build your consumption of specific supplements during these times.

-Occasional changes: Our dietary requirements can change with the seasons, as our bodies might require various supplements to adapt to changes in temperature and openness to the sun.

-Feelings of anxiety: Elevated degrees of stress can affect our skin wellbeing and our bodies might require various supplements to adapt to stress.

-Prescriptions: Certain meds can influence your skin wellbeing and dietary requirements, like oral contraceptives or anti-infection agents.

It's vital to pay attention to your body and make acclimations to your eating routine on a case by case basis. On the off chance that you are encountering skin issues, it's ideal to talk with a dermatologist or nutritionist, who can assist you with deciding the best eating regimen for your particular necessities and objectives.

Taking everything into account, paying attention to your body and changing your eating regimen depending on the situation is significant for keeping up with ideal skin wellbeing. It's essential to make changes on a case by case basis to help ideal skin wellbeing.

# Sleep

Rest expects a basic part in staying aware of sound skin. The following are a couple of inspirations driving why:

- Cell restoration:
During rest, our bodies are endeavoring to fix and re-energize our skin cells, which helps with keeping our skin looking lively and stimulated.

- Disturbance reduction:
Rest helps with decreasing aggravation in the body, which can help with reducing redness, broadening, and breakouts in the skin.

- Hormonal balance:
Rest helps with overseeing synthetic substances, for instance, cortisol and melatonin, which expect a key part in skin prosperity. Raised cortisol levels, for example, can incite extended exacerbation and breakouts.

- Hydration:

Rest helps with hydrating the skin, as our bodies are conveying more hydration-propelling synthetic compounds while we rest.

- Stress decline:

Rest helps with lessening sensations of nervousness, which can be a main issue in skin issues, similar to breakouts and developing.

All things considered, rest expects a fundamental part in staying aware of sound skin. Rest is a key piece of any skin wellbeing management plan. Aim high extended lengths of significant worth rest every night to help ideal skin prosperity.

## Ways to improve sleep

Developing rest quality is significant for keeping up with solid skin and generally speaking wellbeing. Here are a few proposals for further developing rest quality:

#1. Lay out a reliable rest plan: Attempt to hit the hay and wake up simultaneously consistently, even at the end of the week, to lay out a predictable rest design.

#2. Establish a rest favorable climate: Ensure your dozing climate is cool, dull, calm, and agreeable. Consider utilizing shut down draperies, an eye cover, and earplugs to establish a rest favorable climate.

#3. Limit screen time before sleep time: The blue light discharged by electronic gadgets can disturb the creation of melatonin, the chemical that controls rest. Attempt to restrict screen time for essentially an hour prior to sleep time.

#4. Keep away from caffeine, nicotine, and liquor before sleep time: These substances can slow down rest quality and make it harder to fall and stay unconscious.

#5. Work-out routinely: Customary actual work can further develop rest quality and assist you with nodding off quicker. In any case, stay away from overwhelming activity before sleep time, as this can make it harder to nod off.

#6. Unwind before sleep time: Participate in loosening up exercises, like perusing a book, washing up, or rehearsing care, before sleep time to quiet the brain and body and plan for rest.

#7. Address rest issues: On the off chance that you are experiencing difficulty dozing, it's critical to address the basic reason, like rest apnea or sleep deprivation. Talk with a medical care supplier to decide the best game-plan.

## Sleep issues

Tending to rest issues, like a sleeping disorder, is vital for keeping up with sound skin and generally speaking wellbeing. While there are numerous self improvement procedures you can use to further develop rest quality, now and again rest issues continue to happen notwithstanding our earnest attempts. In these cases, looking for proficient help is significant. Here are a few justifications for why:

-Fundamental causes: Rest issues can have basic causes, like rest apnea, a propensity to fidget, or uneasiness, that should be addressed to further develop rest quality. A medical services proficient can assist with diagnosing these fundamental causes and foster a suitable therapy plan.

-Meds: at times, rest issues can be treated with prescriptions, like narcotics or hypnotics. A medical care proficient can decide whether these meds are proper for yourself and screen their utilization to guarantee they are protected and powerful.

-Cognitive based therapy: Cognitive based therapy (CBT) is a kind of treatment that can assist with further developing rest quality by addressing negative contemplations and ways of behaving that add to rest issues. A prepared specialist can help you recognize and address these contemplations and ways of behaving to further develop rest quality.

-Customized approach: A medical services proficient person can give a customized way to deal with further developing rest quality in view of your singular requirements and conditions. They can consider your rest history, way of life, and wellbeing status to foster a methodology that is custom-made to your particular necessities.

Taking everything into account, in the event that you are battling with rest issues, for example, a sleeping disorder, looking for proficient help is significant. By working with a medical care proficient, you can get a customized way to deal with further developing rest quality, address basic causes, think about drug choices, and take advantage of CBT to further develop rest quality and back ideal skin wellbeing.

# Stress management

Stress can altogether affect both aging and skin wellbeing. Here are a few different ways that stress can influence the skin:

<u>Ongoing stress</u>:
Persistent stress can set off the arrival of cortisol, a chemical that can separate collagen, a protein that keeps skin firm and flexible. This can prompt kinks and list skin.

<u>Skin inflammation breakouts</u>: Stress can likewise set off the arrival of chemicals that can cause skin inflammation breakouts. Stress-initiated skin break out can be challenging to treat and can leave scars that can influence the presence of the skin.

<u>Dermatitis</u>:
Stress can likewise set off dermatitis, a skin condition that causes red, irritated, and layered skin. Stress-initiated dermatitis can be hard to

treat and can leave scars that can influence the presence of the skin.

Rosacea:
Stress can likewise set off rosacea, a skin condition that causes redness, flushing, and pimple-like knocks on the face. Stress-initiated rosacea can be challenging to treat and can influence the presence of the skin.

All in all, diminishing stress is significant for keeping up with sound skin. Here are ways to lessen stress:

-Work out: Exercise can assist with decreasing stress by delivering endorphins, which are normal temperament supporters. Exercise can likewise assist with lessening cortisol levels.

-Unwinding methods: Unwinding procedures, like reflection, yoga, and profound breathing, can assist with decreasing stress and advance a feeling of quiet.

-Get sufficient rest: Getting sufficient rest can assist with diminishing stress by giving your body time to fix and recover.

-Eat a solid eating regimen: Eating a sound eating regimen that is wealthy in supplements and cell reinforcements can assist with diminishing stress and further develop skin wellbeing.

Integrating these stress decreasing procedures into your day to day schedule can assist with further developing skin wellbeing, dial back the aging system, and advance in general prosperity.

## Techniques for managing stress

Here are a few procedures for overseeing stress:

- Work out:

Exercise can assist with diminishing stress by delivering endorphins, which are normal state of mind sponsors. Exercise can likewise assist with decreasing cortisol levels.

- Unwinding procedures:

Unwinding methods, like reflection, yoga, profound breathing, and moderate muscle unwinding, can assist with lessening stress and advance a feeling of quiet.

- Care:

Care is the act of being available at the time and focusing on your viewpoints and sentiments without judgment. This can assist with decreasing stress and advance prosperity.

- Using time effectively:

Focusing on your undertakings, laying out reasonable objectives, and assigning liabilities can assist with decreasing stress and further develop efficiency.

- Rest:

Getting sufficient rest can assist with decreasing stress by giving your body time to fix and recover.

- Nourishment:

Eating a sound eating regimen that is wealthy in supplements and cell reinforcements can assist with lessening stress and work on generally wellbeing.

- Look for help:

Conversing with companions, family, or a psychological wellness expert can assist with diminishing stress and offer help during testing times.

- Leisure activities and interests:

Participating in side interests and interests that give you pleasure and unwinding can assist with lessening stress and advance prosperity.

These strategies can be integrated into your day to day everyday practice to assist you with overseeing stress and advance by and large prosperity. Try to find the methods that turn out best for yourself and make them an ordinary piece of your stress the executives schedule.

## How to balance stress in your schedules

Tracking down a balance between overseeing stress and dealing with oneself is significant for keeping up with generally well being and prosperity, including skin wellbeing. At the point when we experience stress, our bodies produce cortisol, a chemical that can adversely affect the skin, including skin inflammation, kinks, and hyperpigmentation.

Integrating stress management procedures into your day to day daily schedule, like activity, unwinding, care, and social help, can assist with lessening feelings of anxiety and advance by and large prosperity. Notwithstanding, it is likewise vital to focus on taking care of oneself exercises, like enjoying reprieves, participating in leisure activities, and getting sufficient rest, to keep a good arrangement.

It is vital to pay attention to your body and perceive when you really want to make a stride back from stress prompting exercises to focus on taking care of oneself. Tracking down a good overall arrangement between overseeing stress and dealing with oneself can assist with advancing solid skin and generally speaking prosperity.

# Makeup and grooming

Picking the right items and apparatuses for cosmetics and prepping is significant because of multiple factors:

**Skin similarity**:
Choosing items that are reasonable for your skin type and responsiveness assists with lessening the gamble of skin bothering, breakouts, and other unfavorable responses.

**Adequacy**:
Utilizing items that are explicitly intended to address your exceptional skincare needs can assist with upgrading the viability of your skincare routine and work on the general wellbeing and presence of your skin.

**Quality**:
Utilizing excellent items that contain top notch fixings can assist with safeguarding and feed

your skin, decreasing the gamble of harm from openness to ecological contaminations.

**Apparatuses**:
Utilizing the right devices, like brushes and wipes, can assist with upgrading the application and in general the look of your cosmetics, as well as decrease the gamble of skin aggravation.

While picking items and devices, it is essential to consider factors, for example, skin type, skin concerns, and individual inclinations, as well as to think about the fixings and nature of the items. Moreover, looking for proficient counsel, like a meeting with a dermatologist or esthetician, can assist you with deciding the best items and instruments for your singular necessities.

Utilizing the right items and apparatuses can assist with improving your cosmetics and preparing schedule, while advancing the general wellbeing and presence of your skin.

# Recommendations when picking cosmetics

While picking cosmetics and makeup items, it is critical to consider factors, for example, skin type, skin concerns, and individual inclinations, as well as to think about the fixings and nature of the items.

Here are a few general proposals for cosmetics and prepping items:

-Cleaning agent: Pick a delicate, pH-adjusted chemical that is reasonable for your skin type and eliminates pollutants without stripping the skin of its normal oils.

-Cream: Select a lotion that is reasonable for your skin type and contains fixings that sustain and hydrate the skin, like glycerin, hyaluronic corrosive, or ceramides.

-Sunscreen: Utilize a wide range sunscreen with basically SPF 30 to shield the skin from destructive UV beams and lessen the gamble of sun harm and skin aging.

-Cosmetics: Pick cosmetics items that are non-comedogenic and liberated from fixings that can aggravate the skin, like scents and parabens.

-Brushes and wipes: Utilize great brushes and wipes to put on your cosmetics, as they can assist with upgrading the application and generally look at your cosmetics while diminishing the gamble of skin disturbance.

-Preparing apparatuses: Pick prepping devices, for example, razors and trimmers, that are delicate on the skin and intended to limit the gamble of skin aggravation and scratches.

It is likewise essential to think about the fixings in the items and pick items that are liberated from hurtful synthetics and substances, for example, parabens, phthalates, and sulfates.

Notwithstanding these suggestions, it is likewise vital to test new items and to look for proficient guidance, like an interview with a dermatologist or esthetician, to decide the best items for your singular requirements.

## Tips for maintaining healthy hair, nails, and skin

Keeping up with sound hair, nails, and skin requires a mix of good sustenance, legitimate skincare, and solid way of lifestyle habits. Here are a few hints to help you accomplish and keep up with solid hair, nails, and skin:

-Nourishment: Eat a fair eating routine that is plentiful in nutrients, minerals, and cell reinforcements, like mixed greens, natural products, and nuts. Consider taking a day to day multivitamin to guarantee that you are getting the essential supplements for solid hair, nails, and skin.

-Hydration: Drink a lot of water to hydrate the skin and advance sound hair and nail development.

-Skincare: Foster a day to day skincare schedule that is custom-made to your singular skin type and concerns, and utilize great items that are liberated from hurtful synthetics and fixings.

-Work out: Integrate ordinary activity into your daily practice to further develop blood stream and oxygenation to the skin, hair, and nails.

-Rest: Get sufficient rest every night to permit the body to recover and fix itself. Go for long stretches of rest each evening.

-Stress management: Practice stress management methods, like yoga, reflection, or profound breathing, to lessen the impacts of weight on the body.

-Stay away from unsafe style habits: Stay away from style habits that can be hurtful to the skin, like smoking, unreasonable sun openness, and inordinate liquor utilization.

-Normal preparation: Routinely groom hair, nails, and skin to keep them looking and feeling amazing. This might involve a profound molding treatment for hair, applying fingernail skin oil to nails, and utilizing peeling cleans for the skin.

-Proficient medicines: Think about proficient medicines, for example, facials, hair shading, and nail medicines, to further improve the wellbeing and presence of your hair, nails, and skin.

Keep in mind, everybody's skin, hair, and nails are unique, and what works for one individual may not work for another. It is essential to pay attention to your body and change your daily practice depending on the situation to accomplish and keep up with solid hair, nails, and skin.

# Lifestyle habits on skin wellbeing and aging

Lifestyle habits can fundamentally affect skin wellbeing and aging. Here are a portion of the manners in which that way of lifestyle habits can influence the skin:

1. Smoking:
Smoking can cause untimely aging and wrinkles due the narrowing of veins in the skin, which can restrict the conveyance of oxygen and supplements to the skin.

2. Sun openness: Delayed sun openness without appropriate security can cause sun harm, including burns from the sun, hyperpigmentation, and an expanded gamble of skin disease.

3. Liquor utilization: Unreasonable liquor utilization can dry out the skin and add to untimely aging.

4. Terrible eating routine: An eating regimen that is deficient in nutrients and supplements can bring about dry, dull, and dormant skin.

5. Absence of rest: Not getting sufficient rest can prompt a lessening in collagen creation and an expansion in irritation, the two of which can add to aging and skin issues.

6. Stress: Persistent stress can increment cortisol levels in the body, which can prompt skin breakouts, wrinkles, and a diminished capacity to mend.

7. Absence of activity: Standard activity is significant for keeping up with sound skin by expanding blood stream and oxygenation to the skin.

By keeping a sound way of life, including legitimate skincare, diet, exercise, and rest style habits, you can assist with decreasing the effect of aging and keep up with solid, energetic looking skin.

## Better lifestyle habits

Here are a few suggestions for better way of lifestyle habits that can assist with further developing skin wellbeing and decrease the impacts of aging:

-Satisfactory rest: Plan to get no less than 7-8 hours of rest every evening and lay out a predictable rest schedule.

-Sound eating routine: Integrate a lot of natural products, vegetables, and entire grains into your eating routine, and break point processed food sources, sugar, and liquor.

-Hydration: Drink a lot of water over the course of the day to keep your skin hydrated.

-Work out: Integrate active work into your everyday daily practice, like a lively walk or yoga, to further develop dissemination and oxygenation to the skin.

-Sun protection: Wear an expansive range sunscreen with a SPF of no less than 30 and breaking point sun openness, particularly between the long stretches of 10 AM and 4 PM when the sun is at its most grounded.

-Stress management: Practice stress diminishing strategies, like contemplation, profound breathing, or actual activity, to lessen cortisol levels and keep up with skin wellbeing.

-Abstain from smoking: Smoking is unsafe to your general wellbeing and can cause untimely aging of the skin.

-Legitimate skincare: Lay out an everyday skincare schedule that incorporates purifying, saturating, and security, and use items that are reasonable for your skin type.

By integrating these style habits into your way of life, you can assist with keeping up with solid, energetic looking skin and diminish the effect of aging.

## Tips for taking care of yourself and living life to the fullest

Tracking down a balance between dealing with oneself and carrying on with life to the fullest is significant for in general prosperity and skin wellbeing. Here are a few motivations behind why:

Stay balanced:
Dealing with yourself and participating in taking care of oneself practices can help forestall burnout, which can adversely affect your skin and by and large wellbeing.

Keep up with psychological wellness:

A fair way of life that incorporates time for unwinding and delight can assist with further developing state of mind and lessen stress, which can decidedly affect skin wellbeing.

Solid style habits:
Participating in sound style habits, like ordinary activity, a reasonable eating routine, and satisfactory rest, can assist with keeping up with skin wellbeing and diminish the impacts of aging.

Satisfaction:
Making every second count, whether through movement, associating, or chasing after side interests, can give joy and satisfaction, which can emphatically affect skin wellbeing and in general prosperity.

It means quite a bit to track down a balance between dealing with oneself and getting a charge out of life, as both are fundamental for generally speaking wellbeing and joy. By dealing with your skin and participating in sound style habits, you can partake in the advantages of looking and feeling your best, while additionally making every second count.

# Encouragement for readers to adopt a healthy happy lifestyle

Embracing a sound and blissful way of life is a fulfilling and satisfying excursion that can carry endless advantages to your skin, brain, and body. Here are a few motivations to urge perusers to take the jump:

- Certainty:

Dealing with your skin and keeping a sound way of life can help certainty and confidence, causing you to feel more content with yourself.

- Expanded Energy:

A solid way of life that incorporates normal activity, a decent eating regimen, and sufficient rest can increment energy levels, permitting you to be more useful and appreciate life without limit.

- Mindfulness:

Taking part in taking care of oneself pursues and embracing better routines can further develop mind-set, diminishing the effect of stress and nervousness on your skin and generally speaking prosperity.

- Long haul benefits:

By dealing with your skin and taking part in solid lifestyle habits, you can partake in the drawn out advantages of looking and feeling your best, very much into your later years.

By embracing a solid, blissful way of life, you can partake in the various advantages that accompany dealing with yourself and your skin. So why pause? Begin your excursion today and find the positive effect it can have on your life!

# Summary

**Skin health management**:

a. Purify your skin two times per day utilizing a delicate cleaning agent to eliminate soil, oil, and cosmetics.

b. Utilize a toner to adjust your skin's pH and set it up for saturating.

c. Apply a cream with SPF consistently, particularly while you will be in the sun.

d. Use eye cream to hydrate and lessen the presence of dark circles and barely recognizable differences.

e. Treat explicit skin concerns, like skin break out or hyperpigmentation, with items that are customized to your requirements.

f. Think about proficient medicines, like facials or compound strips, to help the wellbeing and presence of your skin.

**Work out**:

a. Integrate cardiovascular activities, like running or cycling, into your daily schedule to further develop flow and lift oxygenation to your skin.

b. Integrate strength preparing works out, for example, weightlifting or obstruction and works out, to assemble muscle and consume fat.

c. Take part in proactive tasks that you appreciate, like climbing or swimming, to remain dynamic and spurred.

d. Stretch routinely to increment adaptability, diminish muscle stress, and forestall injury.

**Diet**:

a. Eat a decent eating regimen that incorporates a lot of natural products, vegetables, lean protein, and entire grains.

b. Limit your admission of handled food sources, added sugars, and immersed fats.

c. Remain hydrated by drinking a lot of water and eating food varieties that are high in water content, like watermelon or cucumber.

d. Think about taking enhancements that help solid skin, like biotin, L-ascorbic acid, or Omega-3 unsaturated fats.

e. Pick food sources that are high in cancer prevention agents, like berries, green tea, and dull chocolate, to safeguard your skin from free extreme harm.

**Rest**:

a. Go for the gold nine hours of rest each night to give your skin time to fix and revive.

b. Establish a rest favorable climate by keeping your room cool, dim, and calm.

c. Lay out a loosening up sleep time normal, like perusing or scrubbing down, to set up your body and brain for rest.

d. Stay away from screens, like telephones or TVs, for essentially an hour prior to bed to lessen openness to blue light.

e. Try not to polish off caffeine or liquor before bed, as they can upset your rest quality.

**Stress management**:

a. Practice care and unwinding strategies, like profound breathing or reflection, to diminish stress and advance internal balance.

b. Take part in proactive tasks, like yoga or kendo, to decrease stress and work on physical and mental prosperity.

c. Interface with loved ones, join a club or gathering, or elect to keep up with social connections and encouraging groups of people.

d. Track down solid methods for dealing with especially difficult times, like writing in a diary or rehearsing appreciation, to oversee stress and pessimistic feelings.

e. Look for proficient assistance, like treatment or directing, if important to address industrious stress or emotional well-being issues.

**Cosmetics and Prepping**:

a. Pick cosmetics and prepping items that are delicate and non-aggravating, particularly assuming you have touchy skin.

b. Utilize regular and natural items at whatever point conceivable to limit openness to synthetic substances and hurtful fixings.

c. Try different things with various styles and hope to find what compliments your face shape and elements.

d. Seek customary hair styles and medicines, like profound molding or keratin medicines, to keep your hair solid and gleaming.

e. Deal with your nails by keeping them managed and very much saturated to stay away from dryness, breaking, or weakness.

f. Put resources into great quality cosmetics brushes and instruments, like wipes or magnificence blenders, to assist you with putting on cosmetics easily and equally.

g. Abstain from over-styling your hair, like utilizing exorbitant intensity or synthetics, to forestall harm and breakage.

h. Utilize delicate, sans sulfate shampoos and conditioners to keep your hair and scalp solid and hydrated.

**Lifestyle**:

a. Try not to smoke and restrict liquor utilization, as they can harm your skin and add to the aging system.

b. Wear sun protection, like caps, shades, or sunscreen, while you will be in the sun for broadened timeframes.

c. Get customary check-ups and screenings, for example, yearly physicals or skin disease screenings, to keep up with by and large wellbeing and distinguish any issues almost immediately.

d. Stay away from stress, for example, over-committing or assuming an excess of liability, to lessen stress and work on in general prosperity.

e. Remain genuinely dynamic and take part in relaxation exercises that you appreciate, like cultivating or photography, to remain connected with and satisfied.

**Ecological elements**:
a. Keep a perfect and safe living climate.
b. Limit openness to poisons and contaminations.
c. Remain informed about natural wellbeing dangers and do whatever it may take to lessen your openness to them.
d. Use eco-accommodating items and decrease squander whenever the situation allows.

By following these tips and making them a piece of your everyday daily practice, you can look and feel 30 years more youthful, work on your general wellbeing, and carry on with a blissful and satisfying life.